14-Day Gree Fat Burning Plan:

29+ Powerful Recipes That Rapidly Melts Away Fat, Detoxifies The Body & Boost Your Energy Levels!

KELLIE MCBRIDE

COPYRIGHT © 2014

ALL RIGHTS RESERVED

"By cleansing your body on a regular basis and eliminating as many toxins as possible from your environment, your body can begin to heal itself, prevent disease, and become **STRONGER** and more resilient then you ever dreamed possible"

-The Global Healing Center

DISCLAIMER

No part of this eBook can be transmitted or reproduced in any form including print, electronic, photocopying, scanning, mechanical or recording without prior written permission from the author.

While the author has taken utmost efforts to ensure the accuracy of the written content, all readers are advised to follow the information mentioned herein at their own risk. The author cannot be held responsible for any personal or commercial damage caused by misinterpretation of information.

All ideas, views and thoughts expressed in this eBook are the author's own. References have been provided wherever possible. *14-Day Green Smoothie* is not affiliated, authorized or endorsed with any of the brands and names mentioned in here unless specified otherwise. This book is not meant for promotional or advertising purposes.

All information contained here is meant to be taken as a guideline. The experience can be different from person to person owing to different body types, ingredients, exercise, medical condition; etc the advice contained herein is mentioned in a neutral manner. It is understood that the reader claims responsibility for their own actions.

The author does not claim nor was any guarantee made regarding any success through this book. Therefore they cannot be held responsible should any losses, risks, liabilities or damages occur, that might be linked, directly or indirectly, with the information contained within this book. Please consult with your doctor.

Table of Contents

WHAT ARE GREEN SMOOTHIES? 7

ARE GREEN SMOOTHIES SAFE? 12

   Preparing Yourself For Detoxing 15

CHOOSING THE RIGHT SMOOTHIE BLENDER 18

CAN GREEN SMOOTHIES HELP WITH WEIGHT LOSS? 21

GREEN SMOOTHIE TIPS FOR BEGINNERS 24

   Other Benefits of Green Smoothies 28

30 DETOX RECIPES THAT WILL TRANSFORM YOUR LIFE 32

BREAKFAST SMOOTHIE RECIPES 33

   The Complete Breakfast Smoothie 34

   Detox Breakfast in a Glass 36

   A Berry Beautiful Breakfast Smoothie 38

   Green Overload 40

   The Sicilian Smoothie Delight 42

   Blueberry-Almond-Ginger Smoothie 44

   Lean-Mean-Green Smoothie Machine 46

   Rehydrating Green Smoothie 48

   Carrot, Mango, and Herb Smoothie 50

   Mango-and-Coconut Water Shake 52

LUNCH SMOOTHIE RECIPES 54

   The Super Green Smoothie 55

   Antioxidant Overload 57

   A Super Kale-Fragilistic Green Smoothie 59

   Smells Like Sweet Spirit 62

Alkaline Heaven *64*
Green Strawberry Shake *66*
Wheatgrass and Berry Smoothie *68*
Minty Fresh Apple Smoothie *69*
Nutrilicious Spinach-Pumpkin-Cucumber Smoothie *72*
The "Fat Buster" *74*

DINNER SMOOTHIE RECIPES **76**
The Xena Warrior Tonic *77*
Blissfully Alkaline and Seductively Green *79*
Liver Cleansing Green Smoothie *81*
Smooth and Silky Green Smoothie *83*
Goodness Gracious Juice O'Health *85*
Greens Galore *87*
Lemon-and-Blueberry Tonic *88*
Sensual and Seductive Detox Spirit *90*
Berry Bounty Green Smoothie *92*
Cranberry Crusade *93*

THE 14-DAY FAT BURNING GREEN SMOOTHIE PLAN **95**

CONCLUSION **98**

WHAT ARE GREEN SMOOTHIES?

"All theory, dear friend, is gray, but the golden tree of life springs **ever green."** This quote from Johann Wolfgang von Goethe, famed German writer and politician, poetically describes the meaning behind green smoothies. We all know what smoothies are; they are awesome healthy drinks, primarily blended from fresh fruits and vegetables and are full of vitamins, minerals and sugar and spice and everything nice.

Okay, maybe not sugar and spice all the time but the "everything nice" part certainly qualifies. From there, you only need to color the smoothie "green" by infusing it with green ingredients such as green leafy vegetables and you get something that is so much more valuable – smoothies that bring forth life, drinks that are so much more nutritious than your typical smoothie!

This is where the secret behind the current green smoothie revolution lies. Green smoothies aren't just a fad; green smoothies are thriving not only because everyone is currently drinking something green and people want to copy what others are doing. The truth is that there are many consumers who can passionately attest to the effectiveness of green smoothies in delivering many health benefits ranging from weight loss to detoxification. The reason why green smoothies are all the rage these days is because green smoothies really are magical elixirs of life offering a wide array of nutritional benefits that can cater to one's daily nutritional needs.

So in the technical and literal sense and based on the prevailing norms today, green smoothies are smoothies that are naturally green in color due to the ingredients specifically chosen for blending it. The most common include superfoods and greens like chard, kale, spinach, alfalfa sprouts, broccoli, brussels sprouts, collard greens, chlorella, spirulina and many others. This is an essential distinction that has to be considered if you plan to pursue a green smoothie-based diet; your smoothie recipes have to contain ingredients that are packed with nutrients that they can be naturally considered healthy for you...

And of course, they have to be naturally green. Now, this leads to the second important consideration with green smoothies: the greenest of green drinks are actually an acquired taste. Not everyone automatically falls in love with the green in green smoothies! Fruit shakes, for example, are more widely embraced but green?

Even the green tea latte that is sold in Starbucks has many cringing in fear. The taste is actually one of the biggest reasons why not everyone is eagerly jumping on the green smoothie bandwagon despite the many health benefits that these drinks offer. Green smoothies are often perceived to be yucky, bland, or slimy. The words "yummy" and green smoothie often do not go together in one sentence unless there's a "NOT" before the yummy.

But there are ways around this! Just as any other recipe can be flavored differently depending on the chef, green smoothies can also be made to suit your taste and preferences. We'll talk about this more in the next section but for now, kindly set aside the concept of "perceived taste" and instead focus on what benefits these green smoothies can offer if you are serious with your weight loss detox, and fat burning goals.

This book, therefore, seeks to help you take control of your life by using a concrete smoothies and juicing plan to help you get from where you are now to where you want to go some weeks down the road.

Here's what you can expect to find in this short but concise eBook on green smoothies for detoxing, fat burning and weight loss:

A. A concise discussion about green smoothies, specifically the health benefits, the perceived risks, and what you can do to manage these risks.

B. Tips on how to improve your smoothie-making skills in the kitchen. You don't need to be an expert but if you whip up a great smoothie, you are already halfway home in your struggle to have a delicious and healthy drink.

C. A list of 30 green smoothie recipes that you can use to help you with your fat burning and detox goals.

D. A sample 14-day fat burning plan using the recipes as samples.

E. Enough knowledge to equip you for long-term juicing. What you will learn from this eBook and from the 14-day weight loss and fat burning plan will go a long way towards shaping your strategy for transitioning to a healthier smoothie-based diet and lifestyle.

So, now that we got the basics out of the way, let's get started by answering the most elementary but crucial question.

ARE GREEN SMOOTHIES SAFE?

In a word, YES!

Nobody will argue that green vegetables trump most other foods in terms of nutritional value. Most of the greens used in making smoothies actually have enough vitamin and mineral content to rival tablet and pill supplements on supermarket and pharmacy shelves.

From that alone, you can be confident that green smoothies are safe and, more importantly, beneficial to your health. Of course, this does not come without any caveats. Here are the most important ones.

Over-reliance on green smoothies can lead to a deficiency in certain types of nutrients that are not readily available in plant-based diets. Those who are on vegan diets, for example, are at risk of incurring a deficiency in Vitamin B12, essential fatty acids like Omega-3 and Omega-6, and proteins. These three nutrients remain essential for holistic health and must therefore be replenished by some other means.

Thankfully, we now have many ways to arrest this potential issue. One of the most popular ways to do this is to add nuts into one's diet. Nuts are rich in both proteins and essential fatty acids offsetting the deficiency that happens when one doesn't eat any animal product. For Vitamin B12 deficiency, adding activated yeast for certain green smoothie recipes can also help address the problem.

Over-consumption of oxalate. There is still plenty of debate surrounding the problem of increased oxalate consumption and frankly, it hasn't been fully understood yet.

However, if you want to cover all the relevant bases, it helps to think about oxalate every now and then.

So how do you do this? Well, the most practical approach is to limit your green smoothie routine to within a defined program affecting only a defined period, say the 14 days included in this eBook.

Beyond that, enjoy your greens in moderation and by varying the ways you consume them such as through salads. Washing your greens thoroughly can also help mitigate the oxalate concern. Lastly, you can always have healthy alternatives to green smoothies by, for example, drinking wheatgrass juice instead. Wheatgrass juice is a nutritious drink with low oxalic acid content and that can help you address concerns with high consumption of oxalate in green smoothies.

In addition, you may also think about preparing yourself prior to following a green smoothies detox and fat burning plan such as the one indicated here.

Preparing Yourself For Detoxing

1. Think about your current health and if there's anything you're feeling that can become a potential complication when you start with the detox plan. Ulcers or hyperacidity, for example, can be a source of concern. Diabetes and fluctuating blood sugar levels are another.

   The best approach is always to talk to your doctor first about health conditions that you may have that can lead to adverse reactions when you start implementing this green smoothies detox plan.

   It doesn't matter whether you're just in the home all day or if you are active on campus doing all sorts of extra-curricular and curricular activities; the point is that everyone responds to juicing and smoothies in different ways and you need to have a clear handle of how your body will respond to the demands of a detox plan.

Remember; a detox plan is great for you because it will produce excellent results but you shouldn't be too obsessed with the idea of losing weight and burning fat until you can conclusively say you are healthy enough for detoxing. Your health comes first and everything else comes second.

2. Are you ready for the immediate and medium-term effects of green smoothies? Detoxing is not an easy challenge. When you detox, your body goes through a withdrawal phase where it craves for certain substances that it has gotten used to over the years and failure to take in these substances leads to symptoms like headaches, involuntary muscular twitches or shaking, and even vomiting in certain cases.

When you detox, you are essentially pushing the reboot button but the body isn't able to just reboot on the fly. It needs time to adjust, normalize, re-orient itself, and get used to eating healthy once again.

This period of adjustment is where fat burning and detox plans are made or lost. If you are not mentally and physically ready for the demands, you will have problems that may lead you to abandon the plant. Think about these demands when preparing yourself for the detox plan.

So, are green smoothies safe? Absolutely yes, but safe can only take you as far as what your physical and mental limitations can handle. Think about these for a few minutes before you proceed into the succeeding sections of this eBook.

CHOOSING THE RIGHT SMOOTHIE BLENDER

Choosing the right blending equipment for making smoothies is not that difficult if you know what you are looking for. It really boils down to matching your budget with the quality of the equipment that you need.

High-end blenders, predictably, cost more than average blenders and may deliver fractionally better performance on a day-to-day basis. Again, it depends on what you need and what you're willing to spend in order to get the equipment that closely matches what you want.

So, the most basic question is this: Do you plan to make smoothies as part of your daily diet moving forward or you're not yet sure about how far you can take detoxing and smoothies as a regular routine?

If you're not yet sure, investing in a high-end blender can be a wasted expense. For starters, blenders in the

$80 to $120 range should be sufficient. If, however, you know that you will be making smoothies for a long time, more expensive blenders in the $200 to $300 range should be your primary target.

On the other end, I strongly advise that you avoid those $40 blenders even if you're not yet sure about how your juicing and detoxing lifestyle will progress. Nobody ever had anything good to say about those cheap blenders. And chances are, you'll be replacing those blenders shortly after you bought them, even if you don't use them extensively.

Besides, you will always be able to find some use for a mid-range blender around the house even if you don't detox or juice regularly enough to justify a $100 blender. As a last common, you can never go wrong with three known brands in the market today; the Vitamix, the Blendtec, and the NutriBullet.

These three brands have a long history of being the go-to blenders for personal and commercial applications. If you are at a loss as to what to buy, you can choose from any of these three brands and you should be able to get a dependable and reliable blender that will produce great smoothies every time.

CAN GREEN SMOOTHIES HELP WITH WEIGHT LOSS?

Now that the basic and crucial question has been answered, we go to the core of why this eBook was written in the first place. The question is this: can green smoothies really help you lose weight? If yes, then how? To the first question, the answer is a resounding "Absolutely!"

You are not the first and neither will you be the last person to actually lose weight from a green smoothies plan. Many swear by green smoothies and all that they have to offer for weight loss. Dieticians and researchers, medical professionals, and those who actually embraced detox diets using green smoothies have seen firsthand how a good plan can get you from Weight A to Weight B with Weight B definitely being a much smaller number. So, how is this possible?

The prevailing mechanism seems to be two-fold.

A. **First, juicing helps curb your appetite.** The human body is finely tuned to crave for food when it is not properly nourished. It is a defense mechanism that allows us to survive. To turn off that natural tendency, you only need to ensure that the body is properly nourished. When the body constantly gets all the nutrients that it needs, it switches from "cravings" into building and healing itself using the available nutrients. And because green smoothies are extremely nourishing, then you are far more able to say "no" to the food temptations and better able to lose weight more effectively.

B. **Second, detoxing helps your body by cleaning it of unnecessary materials that are hindering its efficiency.** Think of your body as a machine, for example. A machine doesn't perform as well if it is not regularly serviced. After repetitive use, it accumulates grime and soot and grease in certain places and this compromises the machine's performance. The body works in pretty much the same way.

To make it fully efficient, detoxing helps flush out all the toxins and grime out allowing your organs and tissues to absorb all the nutrients from the food you eat. After that, it goes back to the first point where a properly nourished body no longer needs to crave for so much food in order to get the nutrients that it needs.

Consider detoxing, therefore, as your regular maintenance and reboot button. And with a clean body, you can start fresh and begin to re-train it to just eat healthy food options.

GREEN SMOOTHIE TIPS FOR BEGINNERS

This section shouldn't be complicated and long. Even for beginners, green smoothies should be a fairly easy task that requires little kitchen expertise.

However, there are some tips that can indeed help you enjoy making green smoothies all the more. Here are some of the most useful and most important that you should already be mindful during Day 1 of your green smoothie detox plan.

Always Remember To Use Fresh Ingredients

Frozen ingredients are acceptable but only if you are sure that they are properly stored. Poor storage destroys the ingredient and makes it lose valuable nutrients. There is no practical purpose in making smoothies when the ingredients you are using aren't as nutritious. Remember, your smoothie is only as good as the quality of the ingredients that you use.

It Is Not Recommended To Buy A New Blender But A Reputable Brand Goes A Long Way Into Making Great Smoothies

When you don't properly blend your ingredients, you'll easily get huge chunks that can mess up the taste. For example, large chunks of kale leaves can leave a slightly bitter taste that will upset the flavor of the whole drink. Good blenders create more homogenous drinks that you can enjoy better, not to mention quicker because the chopping and blending action is done in a shorter time than if an old and slow blender were to do it. The final message: invest in a good blender particularly when you want to make green smoothies for the long-term.

Be Extra Careful With Artificial Sweeteners

Losing weight boils down to responsible calorie intake and one way to lower the number of calories you consumed is by cutting back on sweets. You won't lose any weight if you load up on sugars all the time. As an alternative, consider healthier options like date honey or natural honey from bees.

Stay Away From Artificial And Synthetic Ingredients

Powders are acceptable but make sure you are buying the genuine product. Synthetic and artificial ingredients defeat the purposes of detoxing because these ingredients introduce a new set of toxins that can mess up your metabolic processes.

Be Liberal When Making Green Smoothies

Experiment. Find flavor profiles that you like. Don't be gun shy. You are only limited by your imagination when it comes to figuring out which ingredients to use when making green smoothies. Kale and strawberry, for example, is an excellent starting point if you want to just discover how to make good drinks from fresh ingredients.

You Can Adjust The Taste Of Any Recipe

There are no set rules for ingredient ratios, just guidelines. If you find any specific recipe to be particularly overwhelming, add more milk or water or fruit to balance the taste and get the flavor that you really want. Detoxing is "detoxing" in the purest sense of the word but it need not be bland and unappealing to the taste.

Other Benefits of Green Smoothies

Aside from weight loss through detoxing and fat burning, what can one expect from drinking green smoothies? There are quite a few other benefits, actually. Here are some of the more impactful benefits that you can expect out of regularly drinking green smoothies.

Green Smoothies Offer More Balanced Nutrition That Is Within Your Control

We've already talked about this in the last few sections but it bears repeating. At the core of human health is proper and balanced nutrition. Smoothies are excellent in this aspect because you know the ingredients that go into every drink so you get what exactly what it is that you feed into your body.

Plus, because making smoothies is super-easy, you can cover a diverse array of ingredients and nutrients by making a few smoothies a day. Green smoothies allow you to take control of your nutrition in ways that are hard to achieve with conventional diets.

Green Smoothies Are Easily Metabolized

Metabolism determines whether or not your body is able to process and take advantage of the nutrients that is fed into it. In the case of solid food, the task is a bit harder because your digestive tract has to break down every food into the smallest components before nutrients are metabolized.

In the case of smoothies, the nutrients are easily absorbed through the stomach walls and the nutrients get passed into the bloodstream for immediate utilization.

Other Green Smoothie Enthusiasts Swear By Its Many Other Benefits

Try reading testimonies on how green smoothie detox plans changed people's lives and you'll find a few recurring themes that may sound small but are actually powerful consequences of a green drink revolution.

People swear that they have more energy when they drink smoothies they improve their moods, more eager to take on daily challenges, suffer from less minor ailments like headaches, heartburn, or even acne. These may sound trivial at first glance but together, they add up to something so much more substantial and empowering.

Green smoothies offer a life-changing lifeline that you can begin to take advantage today by just trying on the recipes below and following the detox plan that is outlined in the subsequent section.

So, without further ado, let's look at 30 simple but powerful detox recipes that you can count on to help guide you through renewal, transformation, detoxification, and re-birth.

30 DETOX RECIPES THAT WILL TRANSFORM YOUR LIFE

Here are 30 healthy green drinks that you can use to kick-start your new green drink habit. We've broken them down into three sections, each for breakfast, lunch and dinner. Try them all so you can get a better feel for what suits your taste.

BREAKFAST SMOOTHIE RECIPES

The following green smoothie recipes are perfect for a morning fixer-upper and are ideal if you want to kick-start your day in the healthiest and most refreshing way possible.

The Complete Breakfast Smoothie

Serving Size: 2 servings

This is a typical sample of a great breakfast smoothie recipe because it ticks many of the boxes when it comes to nutrition but also because it is full of dietary fibers ideal for detox and cleansing.

In addition, the soya yogurt is a great alkalinizing food that counteracts the natural acidity of the stomach to eliminate any upsets in the morning. The addition of pomegranate juice also makes this a great hydrating drink that can fill you up in the morning.

Ingredients:

150g strawberries

½ cup spinach

1 tbsp. spirulina powder

75g raspberries

1 medium banana, peeled

200ml pomegranate juice

4 tbsp. soya yogurt

Directions:

Mix everything in a blender. Enjoy.

Nutritional Information:

Nutrition-wise, most of the ingredients in this recipe pack a lot of nutritional value. The spinach and spirulina powder boosts one's iron intake while also providing protein and a wide array of vitamins, minerals, and carotenoids. The strawberries and raspberries have plenty of antioxidants that can help protect cells from damage.

160 calories, 25 g protein, 34 g carb, 6 g fiber, 0.3 g fat, 0 g sat fat, 70 mg sodium

Detox Breakfast in a Glass

Serving Size: 2 servings

This is a twist of the previous recipe and is meant to demonstrate that changing the ingredients from one recipe to another does not dramatically change the performance of a smoothie if all the basics are still adequately covered.

In this case, we just substituted the pomegranate juice with the more available lemon juice. The effect is the same but the flavor profile can be different. You can experiment to see which ones suit your preference. You can also work exclusively with this recipe if pomegranate juice is hard to come by in your area.

Ingredients:

1 cup water

1 tbsp. flaxseed

1 cup raspberries

1 medium banana

¼ cup spinach

2 tsp. lemon juice

1 cup ice

Directions:

Place all ingredients in the blender in the order above and blend away.

Nutritional Information:

You already know the nutritional value of the spinach from the previous recipe. The substitution of the pomegranate juice with lemon juice makes this recipe far richer in Vitamin C than the original. Potassium in banana and essential fatty acids from flaxseed also give this recipe an added dimension that makes it stand out from the first one.

180 calories, 16 g protein, 22 g carb, 3 g fiber, 1.3 g fat, 0.2 g sat fat, 35 mg sodium

A Berry Beautiful Breakfast Smoothie

Serving Size: 2 servings

This is a great berry-centric smoothie recipe with the kale only as an accent. The taste of berries dominates this recipe and it helps demonstrate that choosing ingredients can be done more liberally without completely losing the idea behind green smoothies.

Here, the kale only provides a light tinge of green but it is the raspberries and cherries that primarily carry the flavor and give this recipe some much needed personality.

Ingredients:

1 cup raspberries

¾ cup almond milk, unsweetened

½ cup kale

¼ cup cherries, pitted

1 ½ tbsp. honey

2 tsp. ginger, finely grated

1 tsp. ground flaxseed

2 tsp. fresh lemon juice

Directions:

Combine all the ingredients in blender and mix until smooth. Use the lemon juice to adjust the taste to your preference.

Nutritional Information:

Raspberries and cherries are rich in antioxidants and ideal for boosting immunity, preventing inflammation, and lowering risk factors for cancer and heart ailments. Cherries are also great for those people who are susceptible to arthritis-type illnesses.

112 cal, 1 g protein, 26 g carb, 3 g fiber, 1.5 g fat, 0 g sat fat, 56 mg sodium

Green Overload

Serving Size: 2 servings

This recipe is designed with "green" in mind. The nutritional value of this recipe is particularly high in terms of iron and antioxidants. Moreover, the inclusion of cucumber in the list of ingredients gives this recipe a refreshing quality ideal for detoxing diets.

Ingredients:

1 large cucumber

1 cup kale

½ cup romaine

2 stalks celery, chopped

1 broccoli stem

1 green apple, cored, quartered

½ lemon, quartered

Directions:

Juice all the ingredients until smooth. Enjoy!

Nutritional Information:

95 cal, 0.3 g protein, 8 g carb, 7 g fiber, 0 g fat, 0 g sat fat, 21 mg sodium

The Sicilian Smoothie Delight

Serving Size: 2 servings

This Sicilian favorite utilizes common everyday ingredients to demonstrate that smoothies need not be fancy to be effective.

In the island of Sicily, for example, all the fresh produce available at the local markets can be juiced in combination with other ingredients to create a simple, earthy, but nutritious green smoothie that works well with a light salad breakfast.

Taste the charms of Sicily with this simple incarnation that speaks to the simplicity of healthy green drinks.

Ingredients:

6 carrots

3 large tomatoes

2 red bell peppers

4 cloves garlic

4 stalks celery

1 cup watercress

1 cup loosely packed spinach

1 red jalapeño, seeded (optional)

Directions:

Juice all the ingredients until smooth. Enjoy!

Nutritional Information:

92 cal, 0.7 g protein, 2 g carb, 5 g fiber, 0 g fat, 0 g sat fat, 37 mg sodium

Blueberry-Almond-Ginger Smoothie

Serving Size: 1 serving

The ginger juice can be bought from many Asian restaurants. It is often sold in powder form and can be prepared just as you would any juice. Almond milk, on the other hand, can be prepared at home by soaking almonds in water overnight and then blending them to extract the juice.

The addition of blueberries and banana tie all the elements together to create a unique-tasting green smoothie that's perfect for early morning risers.

Ingredients:

1 cup almond milk (or soya milk)

¼ cup blueberries

1 cup kale

1 medium banana

3 tbsp. ginger juice

Directions:

Blend all the ingredients together. Enjoy!

Nutritional Information:

88 cal, 5 g protein, 5 g carb, 4 g fiber, 0.2 g fat, 0.1 g sat fat, 44 mg sodium

Lean-Mean-Green Smoothie Machine

Serving Size: 2 servings

This refreshing smoothie is ideal for breakfast because it is packed with nutrients and has no frills when it comes to nutrition. All the ingredients chosen for this recipe all contribute to the overall completeness of the smoothie.

The mango, apple and cucumber make this a filling drink while the barley grass juice powder provides complementary nutrition that augments the value of the fresh fruits used. Overall, this is a simple recipe that demonstrates how different ingredients can work together to create a balanced and hunger-busting morning drink.

Ingredients:

1 green apple, cored

1 tbsp. barley grass juice powder

1 lemon

1 cucumber, peeled

3 leaves of red lettuce

¼ cup mango

10-oz pure water

Directions:

Blend all the ingredients together. Enjoy!

Nutritional Information:

85 cal, 4.3 g protein, 6 g carb, 6 g fiber, 0 g fat, 0 g sat fat, 57 mg sodium

Rehydrating Green Smoothie

Serving Size: 1 serving

This rehydrating green smoothie perfect for detox because it provides ample water that can help cleanse the toxins out of your body. The addition of coconut kefir which is nothing but fermented coconut water also boosts hydration and enhances the electrolyte profile of this smoothie.

If you want a drink that is specifically kind to your skin, this is the drink that you want to be reaching for early in the morning.

Ingredients:

1 cup coconut kefir

½ cup packed flat-leaf parsley

1 cucumber, seeded

1 medium apple, cored

1 tbsp. coconut oil

1 lime, juiced

2 tbsp. fresh mint leaves

Directions:

Blend all the ingredients and enjoy a fresh and morning beverage.

Nutritional Information:

105 cal, 3.2 g protein, 8 g carb, 3 g fiber, 0.8 g fat, 1 g sat fat, 92 mg sodium

Carrot, Mango, and Herb Smoothie

Serving Size: 2 servings

Carrots and mango are prominent ingredients in most smoothies and are often adequate as stand-alone ingredients. In this mix, we combined both and then added various herbs to give the whole drink a light but tangible kick enough to spice up your palate.

The resulting drink isn't overly "green" because there are no heavy leaves to dominate the flavor. Instead, you can still get the flavor of mango and carrots with the slight hint of mint providing contrast and complexity.

Ingredients:

2 cups mango chunks

1 cup carrot juice, freshly pressed

1 cup orange juice, freshly squeezed

¼ cup fresh herbs (mint, tarragon, basil)

Directions:

Combine all ingredients in a blender; blend until smooth.

Nutritional Information:

225 calories; 0 g saturated fat; 0 g unsaturated fat; 0 mg cholesterol; 56 g carbs; 36 mg sodium; 3 g protein; 5 g fiber

Mango-and-Coconut Water Shake

Serving Size: 2 servings

As far as simple green smoothies go, this mango and coconut water mixture is basic but powerful. The detoxing power of this drink mainly comes from the coconut water as it promotes electrolyte balance and hydration.

The spirulina powder is the main green component and its plethora of nutritional value complements the mango and coconut water mixture well. If you are feeling adventurous, there is always cayenne powder to bring the flavor profile to another level of freshness and complexity.

Ingredients:

2 cups ripe mango chunks

3 tbsp. lime juice, freshly squeezed

2 cups coconut water, unsweetened

Pinch of cayenne powder

1 tbsp. spirulina powder

Directions:

Combine all ingredients in a blender. Blend until smooth. Serve immediately.

Nutritional Information:

159 calories; 1 g saturated fat; 0 g unsaturated fat; 0 mg cholesterol; 39 g carbs; 256 mg sodium; 3 g protein; 6 g fiber.

LUNCH SMOOTHIE RECIPES

These recipes are perfect for to accompany your lunch or as afternoon refreshments. Lunch or afternoon green smoothies tend to contain more liquid ingredients and are also lighter than most other smoothie recipes.

The main intention isn't to fill your stomach; rather, it's to complement a light lunch and allow you to hydrate in the middle of the day while also providing balanced nutrition for health, wellness and cleansing.

The Super Green Smoothie

Serving Size: 2 servings

There are no heavy ingredients in this smoothie, just a wave of green ingredients that provide fiber and are complemented by the orange juice which provides a lot of Vitamin C and ample hydration.

Ingredients:

1¼ cups chopped kale leaves

1¼ cups mango chunks

2 medium celery stalks, chopped

1 cup tangerine or orange juice

¼ cup chopped flat-leaf parsley

¼ cup chopped fresh min

Directions:

Combine all the ingredients in a blender and puree until smooth. Serve immediately.

Nutritional Information:

160 cal, 3 g protein, 39 g carbs, 5 g fiber, 0.5 g fat, 0 g sat fat, 56 mg sodium

Antioxidant Overload

Serving Size: 1 serving

It is well-known that most types of berries are rich in antioxidants that help cleanse the body from disease-causing free radicals. Try out this simple recipe to flavor your afternoon refreshments. The lightness of the drink also makes this an ideal partner to a light afternoon snack.

Ingredients:

2 cups mixed berries

1 cup unsweetened pomegranate juice

1 cup kale

1 tbsp. spirulina or moringa powder

water

Directions:

Combine berries, juice, and 1 cup water in a blender; blend until smooth.

Nutritional Information:

130 calories; 0 g saturated fat; 1 g unsaturated fat; 0 mg cholesterol; 34 g carbs; 19 mg sodium; 1.5 g protein; 4 g fiber.

A Super Kale-Fragilistic Green Smoothie

Serving Size: 2 servings

The name of this smoothie says it's all. It's a fitting and wonderful tribute to Mary Poppins' supercalifragilisticexpialidocious expression from the Disney movie of the same name.

This smoothie is fun and well balanced and the ingredients work together to create a mild-tasting smoothie that's perfect as an afternoon relaxing drink whether you're at the office or out on a beach somewhere enjoying your holiday.

Try this drink and experiment with the ginger to find the right level of spice that you like for your green drinks.

Ingredients:

½ medium pear, pitted

¼ medium avocado, pitted

½ cucumber, chopped

½ lemon

¼ cup cilantro

1 cup kale

½ inch ginger, grated

½ cup coconut water

1 scoop protein powder

1 cup water

Directions:

Blend all ingredients. Enjoy!

Nutritional Information:

140 calories; 0 g saturated fat; 0 g unsaturated fat; 0 mg cholesterol; 28 g carbs; 23 mg sodium; 1.1 g protein; 47g fiber.

Smells Like Sweet Spirit

Serving Size: 2 servings

This tribute to rock band Nirvana is less a cocktail and more a healthy green drink but the comparisons mostly come from the richness of the ingredients when blended together.

This is a creamy drink as it gets a little bit of everything from the almond milk, bananas and even the blueberries. Enjoy this delicious and simple green smoothie that appeals to your civilities as a sophisticated smoothie lover.

Ingredients:

½ medium banana, peeled

½ cup blueberries

¼ avocado, pitted

½ cup almond milk

1 tsp. spirulina powder

1 cup water

Directions:

Blend all ingredients. Enjoy!

Nutritional Information:

160 calories; 0.8 g saturated fat; 0.1 g unsaturated fat; 0 mg cholesterol; 34 g carbs; 45 mg sodium; 1.8 g protein; 26g fiber.

Alkaline Heaven

Serving Size: 1 serving

This green smoothie demonstrates that as few as four carefully chosen ingredients can help you create a simple alkalinizing drink that's perfect for helping you get rid all of the stresses away.

Ingredients:

1 cup papaya, chopped, seeded

1 cup coconut kefir

½ lime, juiced

1 tbsp. raw honey

Directions:

Mix all the ingredients together and blend until smooth.

Nutritional Information:

You can also substitute either coconut yogurt or cultured coconut milk if there is no coconut kefir available.

145 calories; 0.8 g saturated fat; 1.4 g unsaturated fat; 0 mg cholesterol; 17 g carbs; 45 mg sodium; 2.3 g protein; 14g fiber.

Green Strawberry Shake

Serving Size: 2 servings

Spinach is a staple in many green smoothies but you can always control its taste and texture by adding something naturally sweet and acidic such as strawberries.

In this recipe, the combination of spinach and strawberries suspended in a creamy non-dairy milk medium makes this drink ideal both as a refreshment beverage but also as a filling alternative to an unhealthy office lunch.

We suggest preparing this drink at home in the morning, packing it into a juice bottle, and popping it into the office refrigerator to chill. Serve cold during lunch time or early afternoon.

Ingredients:

3 cups nondairy milk of your choice

2 cups fresh strawberries

1 tbsp. lemon zest

1 small orange, peeled

1 banana, peeled

1 ½ cups spinach

Directions:

Using a high-speed blender, blend all ingredients until smooth. Serve immediately.

Nutritional Information:

200 calories; 1.6 g saturated fat; 2.2 g unsaturated fat; 0 mg cholesterol; 31 g carbs; 56 mg sodium; 1.2 g protein; 18g fiber.

Wheatgrass and Berry Smoothie

Serving Size: 2 servings

This recipe primarily thrives on its berry content, a definite must-have for all you lady juicers out there who are looking for some much-needed berry flavors into your detox regimen.

The wheatgrass and coconut kefir are just fillers to tie it all together but the main draw is in the antioxidant goodness that this combination of berries has plenty of.

Ingredients:

1 cup coconut kefir water

1 banana

2 shots wheatgrass juice

¼ cup strawberries and blueberries mixture

3 tbsp. goji berries

Directions:

Mix all the ingredients together and blend until smooth.

Nutritional Information:

115 calories; 1.1 g saturated fat; 0.7 g unsaturated fat; 0 mg cholesterol; 14 g carbs; 39 mg sodium; 2 g protein; 13g fiber.

Minty Fresh Apple Smoothie

Serving Size: 2 servings

This minty fresh apple smoothie is a simple but clever play on combining apples and lettuce together into a smoothie.

The lettuce isn't overly dominating and can be easily controlled by varying the amount that you add into the blend. The apple is essentially the core ingredient in this drink, and this recipe demonstrates that even the most common and basic ingredients can be accentuated by carefully selecting ingredients that blend well but do not overpower the main ingredient.

In the case of adding mint, it gives the drink some level of sophistication that makes it worthy for an afternoon break after a tough and stressful day.

Ingredients:

½ green apple, cored

8 fresh mint leaves

3 leaves of green leaf lettuce

10-oz pure water

Directions:

Blend all ingredients. Enjoy!

Nutritional Information:

94 calories; 0 g saturated fat; 0 g unsaturated fat; 0 mg cholesterol; 19 g carbs; 25 mg sodium; 3 g protein; 22g fiber.

Nutrilicious Spinach-Pumpkin-Cucumber Smoothie

Serving Size: 2 servings

This is another refreshing detox drink that takes advantage of the known qualities of spinach and cucumber to produce a simple drink that is rich in nutrients and all the healthy goodness you can ask for in a drink.

The addition of the orange, lemon and pear only serve to add pizzazz to an already-excellent and nutrilicious drink that is sure to become a mainstay in your repertoire of healthy detox green smoothies.

Ingredients:

1 ½ cup baby spinach

½ small cucumber

1 pear, cored

1 lemon, peeled

1 orange, peeled

1 tbsp. pumpkin seeds

2 cups water

Directions:

Blend all ingredients. Enjoy!

Nutritional Information:

102 calories; 0.2 g saturated fat; 1.4 g unsaturated fat; 0 mg cholesterol; 35 g carbs; 16 mg sodium; 5 g protein; 29g fiber.

Pumpkin seeds are well lauded for their fiber, protein and fat content. You can buy packs of pumpkin seeds during the Halloween period that you can then store for consumption for 3 to 4 months afterwards.

The "Fat Buster"

Serving Size: 1 serving

The fat buster takes advantage of the fat-burning properties of carrots, beet, and radish as well as the green goodness of parsley to fuel your detox regimen.

Carrots and beet, in particular, carry a lot of natural sugars that nourish and supply your body with all the energy that it needs while the fiber in parsley and carrots help cleanse your digestive tract.

The addition of garlic with all its antioxidants gives this drink a unique flavor profile that should help you lose the excess weight.

Ingredients:

1 medium red beet

3 medium carrots

1 radish

2 garlic cloves, finely minced

½ cup flat-leaf parsley

Directions:

Juice all the ingredients. Enjoy!

Nutritional Information:

145 calories; 0 g saturated fat; 0 g unsaturated fat; 0 mg cholesterol; 20 g carbs; 23 mg sodium; 4 g protein; 38g fiber.

DINNER SMOOTHIE RECIPES

Smoothie recipes intended for dinner are often designed with two things in mind: a filling drink that packs a lot of nutrients that will last you through the night as well as an eye towards a relaxing and unwinding beverage in the vein of tonics or cocktails.

In these recipes, we paid careful attention to both aspects of green smoothies so your body is readily equipped to continue the fat burning and detox regimen as you soundly sleep through the night so that the following morning, you are poised to continue chipping away at your goal of sustainable and permanent weight loss.

The Xena Warrior Tonic

Serving Size: 1 serving

Following the "tonic" theme we just mentioned in the introduction to dinner smoothie recipes, this drink takes advantage of the harmony between almond milk and cacao nibs to create a base for what is definitely a healthy and fat-busting green drink.

The end-goal here is to create your own version of a healthy Irish cream without the alcohol and the weight-ruining calories. Instead, you have fresh fruits, a touch of oil for essential fats, and an infusion of spirulina or moringa powder for balance and bulk.

Ingredients:

1 cup almond milk

1 tbsp. spirulina or moringa powder

2 tbsp. chia seeds

1 banana, peeled

1 tbsp. coconut oil

2 tbsp. cacao nibs

1 cup ice

Directions:

Blend all ingredients and enjoy! This smoothie is best served cold.

Nutritional Information:

132 calories; 1.3 g saturated fat; 0.9 g unsaturated fat; 0 mg cholesterol; 22 g carbs; 13 mg sodium; 6 g protein; 19g fiber.

Blissfully Alkaline and Seductively Green

Serving Size: 2 servings

This blissfully alkaline drink relies on the pleasant combination of almond milk and coconut water to give you a solid smoothie base that is then given depth by the avocado and spinach.

The protein powder is added to give you a real source of protein to balance your fruit-and-veggie-based diet. Lastly, the chia seeds take advantage of the superfood properties of the chia, providing plenty of vitamins, minerals and fiber for balanced nutrition and thorough cleansing.

Ingredients:

½ medium pear, pitted

¼ avocado, pitted

1 cup spinach

¼ cup coconut water

1 cup almond milk

1 tsp. chia seeds

1 tbsp. whey protein powder

1 cup water

Directions:

Blend all ingredients until smooth and creamy!

Nutritional Information:

154 calories; 0.3 g saturated fat; 0.7 g unsaturated fat; 0 mg cholesterol; 27 g carbs; 48 mg sodium; 18 g protein; 14g fiber.

Liver Cleansing Green Smoothie

Serving Size: 2 servings

This smoothie needs very little introduction. The kale, apple and beet are mainstays in most smoothie recipes.

With its high fiber content, this drink is able to absorb all of the bad cholesterol in your digestive tract allowing for cleansing and giving your liver a much-needed break from fatty diets that leave you feeling bloated and slow.

Ingredients:

2 cups kale

¼ cup parsley

1 small beet, scrubbed, quartered

1 apple, cored

1 lemon, peeled

½ inch fresh ginger, grated

1 tbsp. chia seeds

2 cups water

Directions:

Blend until smooth. Serve immediately.

Nutritional Information:

115 calories; 0 g saturated fat; 0.2 g unsaturated fat; 0 mg cholesterol; 15 g carbs; 23 mg sodium; 8 g protein; 38g fiber.

Smooth and Silky Green Smoothie

Serving Size: 2 servings

This green smoothie epitomizes the true definition of cleansing without having to starve you. The apple, lettuce leaves, avocado and cucumber more than makes for a great dinner.

Blending them together with nutrient-rich spirulina powder and adding protein to that mix will give you an energizing cleansing drink that you can rely on a daily basis to fill your belly but also help you burn the fat.

Ingredients:

5 large romaine lettuce leaves

½ medium apple

¼ avocado, pitted

½ cucumber, chopped

¼ cup cilantro

1 whole lime

3 tbsp. protein powder

2 tbsp. spirulina powder

1 tsp. raw honey

1 cup water

Directions

Blend until smooth. Serve immediately.

Nutritional Information:

170 calories; 0.8 g saturated fat; 2.1 g unsaturated fat; 0.1 mg cholesterol; 22 g carbs; 12 mg sodium; 33 g protein; 16g fiber.

Goodness Gracious Juice O'Health

Serving Size: 2 servings

The addition of blueberries to this otherwise simple drink gives it tons of antioxidants that complement the vitamins, minerals and fiber in kale. The coconut water is also helpful in balancing your electrolytes while the cucumber provides more than enough water to rehydrate your cells.

Ingredients:

1 avocado, pitted

1 banana, peeled

1 cup blueberries

1 cucumber

½ cup kale or romaine or spinach (your choice)

1 cup coconut water

a sprinkle of cinnamon (optional)

Directions:

In a high-speed blender, blend all ingredients until smooth. Serve immediately.

Nutritional Information:

151 calories; 0.7 g saturated fat; 1.3 g unsaturated fat; 0 mg cholesterol; 12 g carbs; 45 mg sodium; 19 g protein; 11g fiber.

Greens Galore

Serving Size: 2 servings

This is the ultimate green drink packing all the important ingredients into one filling and detoxing smoothie that's perfect as dinner in and of itself. You can add more spirulina or chlorella if you want to boost the nutritional value of this smoothie.

Ingredients:

1 cup coconut water

3 stalks kale

¼ cup spinach

½ cup packed flat-leaf parsley

½ cup cilantro

2 green apples

¼ tsp. ginger, freshly grated

1 heaping tbsp. wild blue-green algae (spirulina or chlorella)

Directions:

Blend all ingredients. Enjoy!

Nutritional Information:

84 calories; 0 g saturated fat; 0 g unsaturated fat; 0 mg cholesterol; 15 g carbs; 21 mg sodium; 39 g protein; 24g fiber.

Lemon-and-Blueberry Tonic

Serving Size: 1 serving

Another simple recipe that is packed with antioxidants from the blueberries, fiber from the kale, and copious amounts of Vitamin C from the lemon, this is a great tonic after a tiring day.

The coconut water also ensures that you properly re-hydrate while promoting electrolyte balance and alkalinity.

It also doesn't hurt that there's just 75 calories in every serving of this wonderful drink.

Ingredients:

1 cup alkaline water or coconut water, depending on what's available

1 cup kale

¼ cup blueberries

1 lemon

Directions:

Blend all ingredients. Enjoy!

Nutritional Information:

75 calories; 0 g saturated fat; 0 g unsaturated fat; 0 mg cholesterol; 10 g carbs; 37 mg sodium; 18 g protein; 7g fiber.

Sensual and Seductive Detox Spirit

Serving Size: 2 servings

The cherries in this drink reminds you of a refreshing cocktail drink while the hemp seeds and cacao powder add a unique layer of flavor that transforms this drink to a super enjoyable dinner accompaniment.

Add the spirulina powder to boost the nutritional value of the smoothie and flavor with raw honey or date honey depending on your preference.

Ingredients:

1 tbsp. cacao powder

2 tbsp. hemp seeds

5 red endive leaves

1 tsp. raw honey or date honey

¼ cup of dark red cherries

10-oz pure water

1 cup ice

1 tbsp. spirulina powder

Directions:

Blend all ingredients. Enjoy while still cold!

Nutritional Information:

117 calories; 0 g saturated fat; 0 g unsaturated fat; 0 mg cholesterol; 16 g carbs; 43 mg sodium; 45 g protein; 17g fiber.

Berry Bounty Green Smoothie

Serving Size: 1 serving

This bountiful berry smoothie is light to the taste but heavy in essential nutrients. Make this smoothie if you need a fixer-upper from a very demanding day at work.

Ingredients:

1 cup coconut milk

1 cup blueberries

½ cup raspberries

½ cup blackberries

2 tbsp. goji berries

1 tbsp. coconut oil

1 tbsp. flaxseed, ground

½ cup flat-leaf parsley

2 dates, pitted

Directions:

Mix all the ingredients and blend until smooth.

Nutritional Information:

104 calories; 0.2 g saturated fat; 0.4 g unsaturated fat; 0 mg cholesterol; 16 g carbs; 31 mg sodium; 25 g protein; 14g fiber.

Cranberry Crusade

Serving Size: 1 serving

The main calling card for this recipe is the cranberries. Cranberries are great cocktail additions, much like cherries, and so this drink is a bit on the wild end in terms of providing both detox and kick.

Enjoy this drink as your stand-alone dinner if you want to skip a heavy meal and instead would want to just have a refreshing beverage that allows you to kickback and recharge from a tiring day.

Ingredients:

½ cup cranberries

1 large celery stalk

1 cucumber

1 apple

1 pear

½ cup spinach

Directions:

Juice all the ingredients. Enjoy!

Nutritional Information:

121 calories; 0 g saturated fat; 0 g unsaturated fat; 0 mg cholesterol; 14 g carbs; 35 mg sodium; 25 g protein; 12g fiber.

THE 14-DAY FAT BURNING GREEN SMOOTHIE PLAN

So now we have the recipes; try this fat burning and detox plan to get your cleansing regimen going.

Day	Breakfast	Afternoon	Dinner
1	Green Overload	Antioxidant Overload	Liver Cleansing Green Smoothie
2	The Complete Breakfast Smoothie	Green Strawberry Shake	Smooth and Silky Green Smoothie
3	Mango and Coconut Water Shake	Minty Fresh Apple Smoothie	Blissfully Alkaline and Seductively Green
4	Carrot Mango and Herb Smoothie	Alkaline Heaven	The Xena Warrior Tonic
5	Rehydrating Green	The Super Green Smoothie	Greens Galore
6	Blueberry Almond Ginger	Wheatgrass and Berry Smoothie	Liver Cleansing Green Smoothie

	Smoothie		
7	The Complete Breakfast Smoothie	The Fat Buster	Cranberry Crusade
8	Detox Breakfast in a Glass	Minty Fresh Apple Smoothie	Lemon and Blueberry Tonic
9	Lean Mean Green Smoothie Machine	Super Kale-Fragilistic Green Smoothie	Goodness Gracious Juice o'Health
10	Carrot, Mango, and Herb Smoothie	Nutrilicious Spinach-Pumpkin-Cucumber Smoothie	Blissfully Alkaline and Seductively Green
11	A Berry Beautiful Breakfast Smoothie	Smells Like Sweet Spirit	Smooth and Silky Green Smoothie
12	Green Overload	Alkaline Heaven	Berry Bounty Green Smoothie
13	The Sicilian Smoothie Delight	The Super Green Smoothie	Sensual and Seductive Detox Spirit

| 14 | Rehydrating Green | Green Strawberry Shake | Greens Galore |

CONCLUSION

Green smoothies are great partners for health and wellness. Green smoothies made from a balance of great ingredients are guaranteed to help you burn fat and lose weight by nourishing your body with all the nutrients that it needs in order to function effectively.

To kickstart your juicing habit, you can refer to the 14-day smoothie plan here. Beyond that, you can regularly do detox regimens every 2 to 3 months depending on your preference. In addition, the more you transition to a whole foods diet, the less is your need for a regular detox routine as your diet should be able to take care of nourishing and balancing your body's health needs on a daily basis.

Lastly, always be mindful of the ingredients you use as well as your body's response to your juicing and smoothie fat burning plan. Adjust your regimen accordingly to suit your needs so you can truly enjoy the power of green smoothies for a healthy, lean and strong body. Enjoy, and cheers to a healthy and long life fueled by green smoothies!

Enjoy this book?

Please leave a review below and let us know what you liked about this book by clicking on the Amazon image below.

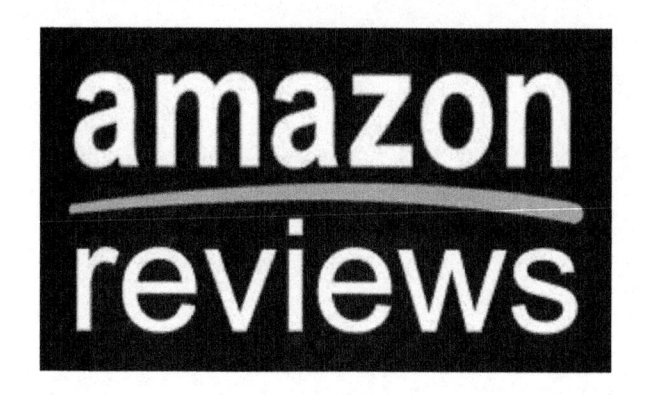

amazon reviews

and click on Digital Orders.

The above link directs to Amazon.com. Please change the .com to your own country extension.

14-DAY GREEN SMOOTHIE

Printed in Great Britain
by Amazon